QUICK AND SIMPLE

WALL PILATES

WORKOUTS

28-day challenge – Illustrated step by step guide to improve your flexibility, posture, mobility, strength and balance for seniors, women and beginners

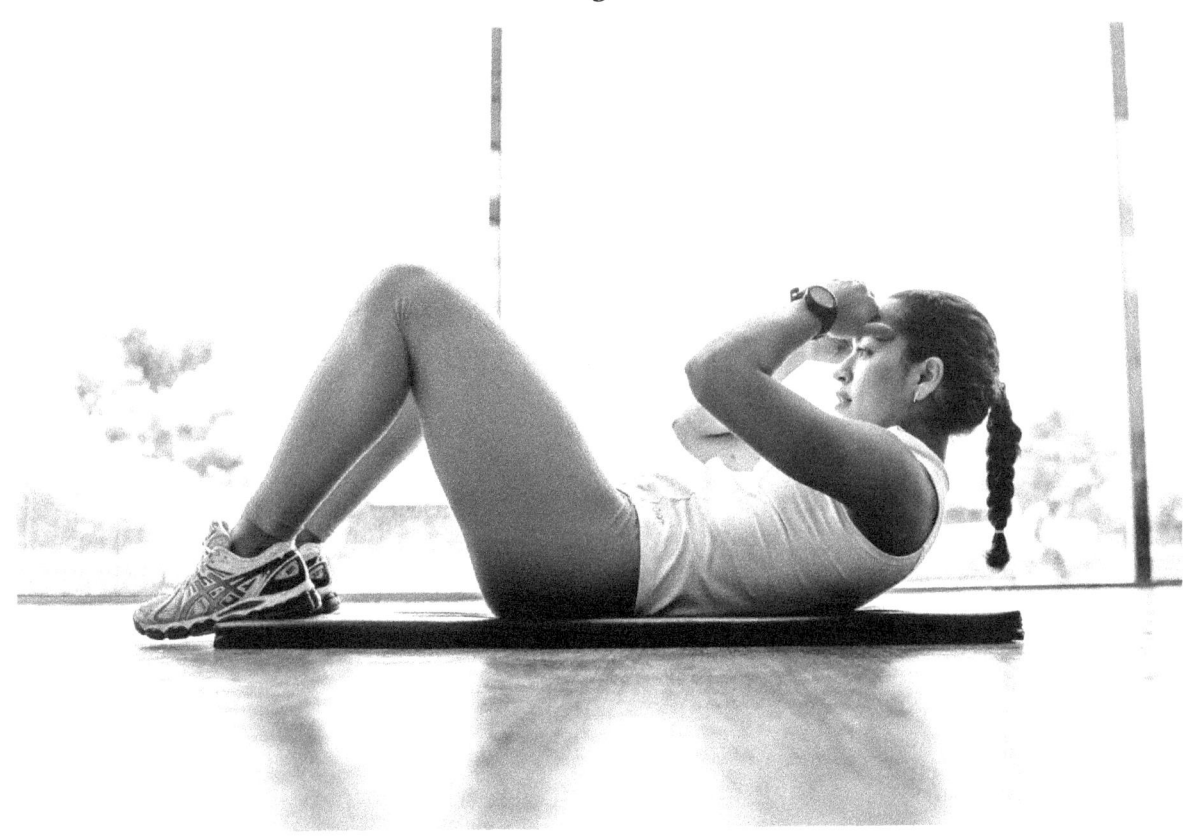

Addison Mitchell

Copyright © [2024] by [Addison Mitchell]

All rights reserved. No part of this publication may be reproduced, distributed, or transmitted in any form or by any means, including photocopying, recording, or other electronic or mechanical methods, without the prior written permission of the publisher, except in the case of brief quotations embodied in critical reviews and certain other noncommercial uses permitted by copyright law.

This book is designed to provide information about Wall Pilates workouts for seniors over 60. The content is intended for educational purposes and is not a substitute for professional medical advice, diagnosis, or treatment. Always seek the advice of your physician or qualified health provider regarding any medical condition or before starting any fitness program.

The author and publisher of this book have made reasonable efforts to ensure the accuracy of the information provided. However, they disclaim responsibility for any liability, loss, or risk, personal or otherwise, which is incurred as a consequence, directly or indirectly, of the use and application of any of the contents of this book.

Any reference to specific exercises, techniques, or nutritional advice is intended for informational purposes only and may not be suitable for every individual. Readers are encouraged to consult with qualified fitness professionals or healthcare providers before initiating any exercise program or dietary changes.

While every effort has been made to provide current and up-to-date information, the author and publisher do not guarantee the accuracy, completeness, or timeliness of the content presented in this book.

About the author: Addison Mitchell

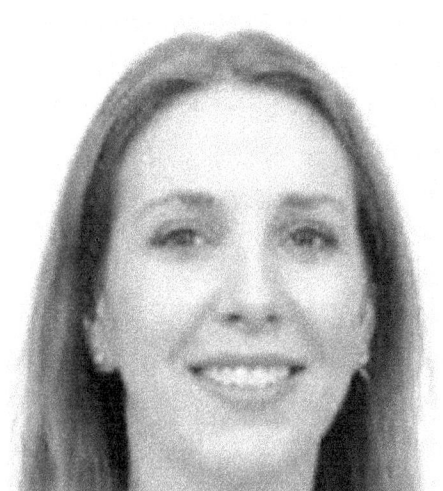

Addison Mitchell is a distinguished authority in the realm of fitness, specializing in an array of disciplines, including workouts, physical training, yoga, and Pilates. With an illustrious career spanning over two decades, Addison has dedicated her life to promoting holistic well-being through her expertise in movement, exercise, and mindful practices.

Expertise and Specializations:

As a seasoned professional, Addison possesses an extensive knowledge base encompassing a diverse spectrum of fitness methodologies. Her proficiency in crafting tailored workout regimens, guiding individuals through transformative physical training sessions, and instilling the principles of yoga and Pilates as foundational aspects of wellness has garnered her widespread acclaim.

Addison's unique approach lies in her ability to fuse the traditional principles of ancient practices like yoga and Pilates with contemporary fitness methodologies. Her programs emphasize not only physical prowess but also mental fortitude, aiming to create a harmonious balance between mind, body, and spirit.

Achievements:

Throughout her career, Addison Mitchell has achieved remarkable milestones and accolades. Her contributions to the fitness industry have been recognized through various awards and commendations. She has been a keynote speaker at prestigious fitness conferences, sharing her expertise and insights with professionals and enthusiasts alike.

Addison's impact extends beyond conventional fitness circles. She has been featured in numerous publications, authored articles on fitness and well-being, and appeared on television shows advocating for a healthier and more active lifestyle.

Her journey:

Addison's journey into the realm of fitness and wellness was not merely a career choice but a profound personal calling. Her passion for movement and its transformative power was ignited during her formative years when she discovered the profound impact of exercise on her own physical and mental well-being.

Driven by an insatiable curiosity and an unwavering dedication to her craft, Addison embarked on a journey of exploration and mastery. She delved into various fitness modalities, honing her skills under the tutelage of renowned mentors and immersing herself in the teachings of ancient practices that eventually became integral to her approach.

With a compassionate heart and a commitment to empowering others, Addison Mitchell embarked on a mission to share her knowledge and expertise. Her desire to help individuals discover their inner strength, achieve optimal health, and embrace holistic wellness has been the cornerstone of her career.

Today, Addison stands as a beacon of inspiration in the fitness world, impacting countless lives through her guidance, teachings, and unwavering dedication to promoting a healthier, more balanced way of life. Her legacy continues to evolve as she remains committed to empowering individuals on their journey to vitality, resilience, and well-being.

TABLE OF CONTENT

About the author: Addison Mitchell.......................... 3

TABLE OF CONTENT 5

Introduction to wall Pilates 11

Overview of Pilates principles 13

Benefits of Wall Pilates 16

Chapter 1: Foundations of Wall Pilates 18

Fundamental Principles 18

Understanding Alignment and Posture in Wall Pilates 18

Breathing Techniques 20

Core Engagement 22

Wall Basics 24

Using the Wall for Support 24

Safety Measures and Precautions 26

Chapter 2: Wall Pilates Exercises............................ 28

1. Wall Squats Variations 28

    1. Basic Wall Squats.. 29

    2. Wall Squats with Leg Raises 29

    3. Wall Squats with Ball Squeeze 30

    4. Wall Squats with Arm Raises 30

    5. One-Legged Wall Squats.. 31

    6. Wall Squats with Resistance Band 32

    7. Dynamic Wall Squats 32

    8. Wall Squats with Calf Raises 33

    9. Wall Squats with Rotation.. 33

    10. Wall Squat Holds with Arm Variations............................... 34

2. Wall Roll-Down Variations 35

    1. Controlled Roll-Downs 35

    2. Roll-Downs with Arm Movements.. 35

    3. Wall Roll-Downs for Flexibility... 36

    4. Roll-Downs with Spinal Twist 37

    5. Wall Roll-Downs with Resistance Band 37

    6. Wall Roll-Downs with Pelvic Tilt... 38

    7. Wall Roll-Downs with Leg Slide 38

    8. Dynamic Wall Roll-Downs... 39

9. Wall Roll-Downs with Arm Circles 40

3. Wall Push-Ups Variations 42

1. Basic Wall Push-Ups 42

2. Decline Wall Push-Ups 42

3. Incline Wall Push-Ups 43

4. One-Arm Wall Push-Ups 43

5. Wall Push-Ups with Shoulder Taps 44

6. Wall Push-Ups with Leg Raises 44

7. Plyometric Wall Push-Ups 45

8. Wall Push-Ups with Resistance Band 46

9. Diamond Wall Push-Ups 46

10. Wall Push-Up Holds 47

4. Wall Angels Variations 48

1. Basic Wall Angels 48

2. Wall Angel Holds 48

3. Dynamic Wall Angels 49

4. Wall Angels with Resistance Band 49

5. One-Arm Wall Angels 50

6. Wall Angel Circles 50

7. Wall Angel Pulses 51

8. Wall Angel Twist 52

9. Wall Angels with Leg Movements 52

10. Wall Angel Flow 53

5. Wall Plank Variations 54

1. Basic Wall Plank 54

2. Wall Plank Holds with Arm Variations 54

3. One-Legged Wall Plank 55

4. Wall Plank with Leg Lifts 55

5. Wall Plank Twists 56

6. Wall Plank with Knee Tucks 57

7. Wall Plank Shoulder Taps 57

8. Wall Plank with Arm Reaches 58

9. Wall Plank with Side Leg Raises 58

10. Wall Plank Flow 59

Chapter 3: Advanced Wall Pilates Workouts 60

Challenging Wall Pilates Sequences 60

1. Wall Pilates Full-Body Flow Sequence 60

2. Advanced Wall Pilates Strength Circuit 61

3. Wall Pilates Dynamic Power Sequence 62

4. Wall Pilates Core and Stability Fusion 63

5. Wall Pilates Advanced Flexibility Sequence 64

6. Wall Pilates Strength and Endurance Fusion 65

7. Dynamic Wall Pilates Core Challenge 66

8. Wall Pilates Functional Strength Circuit 67

9. Wall Pilates Mobility and Flexibility Sequence 68

10. Wall Pilates Dynamic Power and Strength Circuit 69

Progressive Wall Pilates Routines 70

Routine 1: Wall Pilates Foundation 70

Routine 2: Building Stability 71

Routine 3: Increasing Endurance 72

Routine 4: Introducing Complexity 73

Routine 5: Advanced Strength and Control 74

Routine 6: Progressive Flow and Endurance 75

Routine 7: Complex Movements and Balance 76

Routine 8: Advanced Functional Strength 77

Routine 9: Advanced Flexibility and Stability Fusion 78

Routine 10: Advanced Dynamic Power Circuit 79

Chapter 4: Enhancing Your Wall Pilates Practice 80

Mindfulness and Relaxation 80

Incorporating Mindfulness Techniques 81

Cooling Down with Wall Pilates 83

Optimizing Your Wall Pilates Journey 85

Tips for Long-Term Commitment 87

BONUS: 28 DAY CHALLENGE 90

Meet the Author: Addison Mitchell 92

Other works by Addison Mitchell 93

Conclusion 95

Thanking Readers and Contributors 97

Introduction to Wall Pilates

Pilates is a kind of exercise that emphasizes strengthening the muscles in the core, enhancing balance and posture, and enhancing general health. A excellent choice for elders or anyone with restricted mobility, wall Pilates is a modified form of classic Pilates that uses a wall for support.

Joseph Pilates created the Pilates method in the early 1900s as a means of healing for injured troops. It developed into a well-liked workout regimen throughout time for those trying to become fitter overall. In wall Pilates, people may complete movements that would otherwise be difficult or hard since the wall offers a sturdy platform for support.

Wall Pilates has several advantages for older people. Wall Pilates may assist increase stability and balance by strengthening the core muscles, which lowers the danger of falling. It may also lessen stress and anxiety, enhance circulation, and aid with posture and flexibility. Furthermore, Wall Pilates may enhance memory and cognitive function, which makes it a fantastic choice for anyone who want to maintain mental acuity as they age.

A wall and a cozy pair of shoes are all you need to begin practicing wall Pilates. It is crucial to choose a roomy, well-lit space for your exercise and to dress in comfortable, fully-range-of-motion apparel. Make sure to warm up with a few minutes of easy cardio, such walking or gentle stretching, before starting your exercise.

There is no shortage of possibilities when it comes to Wall Pilates exercises. Exercises like wall squats, wall push-ups, wall sit-ups, wall bridges, and wall planks are very common. It's crucial to begin with workouts suitable for your current level of fitness and to progressively increase the challenge as you advance.

The ability to customize Wall Pilates to each person's requirements and skills is one of its many wonderful qualities. Exercises may be done sitting down or with the assistance of a chair for elderly people with restricted mobility.

Modifications to lessen impact and improve comfort may be implemented for those with long-term ailments like arthritis.

To sum up, elders may engage in safe and efficient workout using wall Pilates. It's a fantastic choice for anybody trying to become fitter and keep their independence as they get older because of its emphasis on strengthening the core, enhancing posture and balance, and boosting general wellbeing. Wall Pilates is a workout that seniors who want to remain active and healthy for years to come should definitely undertake due to its numerous advantages.

Overview of Pilates principles

Pilates, developed by Joseph Pilates in the early 20th century, is a holistic approach to physical fitness that emphasizes strength, flexibility, balance, and mind-body connection. Central to the Pilates method are its fundamental principles, serving as the core philosophy guiding every movement and exercise within the practice.

1. Concentration

At the heart of Pilates lies the principle of concentration. Each movement demands focused attention to engage specific muscle groups and maintain proper form. By being fully present in the exercises, practitioners enhance body awareness, refining their movements for maximum effectiveness.

2. Control

Control is the essence of Pilates. Rather than performing exercises rapidly, practitioners emphasize controlled, precise movements executed with deliberate intention. This deliberate control not only ensures safety but also deepens the engagement of targeted muscles, fostering better strength and stability.

3. Centering

The concept of centering in Pilates refers to the body's core, often called the "powerhouse." This area, encompassing the abdominal muscles, lower back, hips, and glutes, serves as the focal point for initiating and stabilizing movements. Strengthening the core is fundamental for overall strength, balance, and posture.

4. Precision

Precision in movement execution is a cornerstone of Pilates. Practitioners strive for accuracy in performing each exercise, emphasizing proper alignment, range of motion, and muscle engagement. Through precise movements, individuals can effectively target specific muscle groups, promoting balanced development and minimizing strain on other areas.

5. Breathing

Breathing techniques in Pilates are integral to enhancing the mind-body connection. The practice advocates for controlled, coordinated breathing that complements movements. Inhaling deeply through the nose to expand the ribcage and exhaling fully through the mouth aids in oxygenating the muscles, enhancing relaxation, and maintaining focus.

6. Flow or Fluidity

Pilates movements are designed to promote a fluid and seamless flow from one exercise to another. Flowing transitions between exercises not only maintain the engagement of targeted muscles but also contribute to the overall grace and efficiency of movement.

Integrating the Principles

These core principles of Pilates are interwoven and interdependent. Practitioners engage in a mindful practice where concentration leads to control, control ensures precision, precision enhances the flow of movements, all supported by centeredness and rhythmic breathing.

Benefits of Pilates Principles for Seniors

For seniors over 60, embracing these Pilates principles offers a multitude of benefits. Enhanced body awareness, improved posture, increased flexibility, and strengthened core muscles contribute to better balance, reduced risk of falls, and enhanced overall well-being. The gentle and controlled nature of Pilates exercises makes it an ideal fitness regimen for seniors seeking to maintain or improve their physical health without placing excessive stress on joints or muscles.

Benefits of Wall Pilates

Wall Pilates offers a multitude of benefits that encompass physical, mental, and even rehabilitative aspects, making it a versatile and holistic fitness practice.

Physical Benefits:

1. **Core Strengthening:** Wall Pilates engages the core muscles profoundly, enhancing stability and strength in the abdomen, back, and pelvis. The wall acts as both support and resistance, intensifying core activation in various exercises.

2. **Improved Posture:** Through alignment-focused movements against the wall, practitioners develop heightened awareness of proper posture. This awareness often translates into better posture in everyday activities, reducing strain on the spine and muscles.

3. **Enhanced Flexibility:** Wall-based exercises promote controlled movements, aiding in stretching and lengthening muscles. The support of the wall allows for deeper stretches, fostering increased flexibility over time.

4. **Increased Strength:** By utilizing the resistance provided by the wall, individuals can build muscular strength in the lower body, upper body, and core. This can contribute to better overall strength and endurance.

5. **Joint Stability:** Wall Pilates exercises, when performed mindfully, contribute to joint stability and mobility. Controlled movements against the wall can aid in strengthening muscles around joints, reducing the risk of injuries.

6. **Balance and Coordination:** Many Wall Pilates movements challenge balance and coordination, improving these aspects through controlled, deliberate exercises performed against the wall.

Mental and Emotional Benefits:

1. **Stress Reduction:** The focus on breathing, mindful movements, and concentration in Wall Pilates can act as a stress reliever, promoting relaxation and mental clarity.

2. **Mind-Body Connection:** Practicing Wall Pilates cultivates a strong mind-body connection. Individuals become more attuned to their bodies, learning to move with intention and awareness.

3. **Increased Energy:** Engaging in regular Wall Pilates workouts can boost energy levels, leaving practitioners feeling invigorated and refreshed.

4. **Enhanced Well-being:** The combination of physical activity, mental focus, and the feeling of accomplishment after a workout can contribute to an overall sense of well-being and positivity.

Rehabilitative Benefits:

1. **Injury Recovery:** Wall Pilates is often used as a part of rehabilitation programs due to its gentle yet effective nature. It can aid in recovering from certain injuries by strengthening muscles without placing excessive strain on the injured area.

2. **Pain Management:** For individuals dealing with chronic pain, Wall Pilates can offer relief by strengthening supportive muscles, improving posture, and promoting better body mechanics.

3. **Preventive Measures:** Regular practice of Wall Pilates can serve as a preventive measure against various musculoskeletal issues by improving strength, flexibility, and alignment.

Overall, the benefits of Wall Pilates extend far beyond physical fitness, encompassing mental well-being and rehabilitative aspects, making it a well-rounded practice for individuals of all fitness levels and ages.

Chapter 1: Foundations of Wall Pilates

Fundamental Principles

Understanding Alignment and Posture in Wall Pilates

Importance of Proper Alignment:

Alignment is the cornerstone of Wall Pilates, focusing on the optimal positioning of the body during exercises. It's about achieving a balanced and efficient posture that minimizes stress on the muscles and joints while maximizing the effectiveness of movements.

1. **Spinal Alignment:** The spine plays a pivotal role in Wall Pilates. Emphasizing a neutral spine position, where the natural curves of the spine are maintained, is fundamental. This alignment supports the core and ensures proper engagement of muscles throughout the practice.

2. **Pelvic Alignment:** Proper pelvic alignment is crucial for stability and optimal muscle engagement. Understanding how the pelvis functions in different exercises against the wall helps in maintaining a strong and stable base.

Principles of Posture in Wall Pilates:

1. **Head and Neck Alignment:** The alignment of the head and neck affects the entire spinal column. Keeping the head in a neutral position, aligned with the spine, prevents unnecessary strain on the neck muscles and supports proper alignment of the rest of the body.

2. **Shoulder and Upper Body Alignment:** Wall Pilates encourages a relaxed yet engaged posture in the shoulders. Proper alignment of the shoulders aids in maintaining stability during exercises against the wall, preventing undue tension in the neck and upper back.

3. **Lower Body Alignment:** Alignment from the hips down to the feet is vital. Wall Pilates exercises often involve proper alignment of the hips, knees, and ankles to ensure stability and prevent injury.

Techniques to Achieve Proper Alignment:

1. **Mindful Awareness:** Wall Pilates places emphasis on mindful movement and body awareness. Practitioners are encouraged to be mindful of their body positioning and make subtle adjustments to achieve optimal alignment during exercises.

2. **Cueing and Visualization:** Instructors often use verbal cues and visualizations to guide participants into correct alignment. These cues help individuals understand and visualize the correct positioning of their bodies against the wall.

3. **Prop Utilization:** Props like mirrors, alignment bars, or even tactile feedback aids (such as small balls placed against the spine) can assist practitioners in understanding and achieving proper alignment while using the wall for support.

Benefits of Proper Alignment and Posture:

1. **Reduced Risk of Injury:** Correct alignment minimizes strain on muscles and joints, reducing the risk of injury during Wall Pilates workouts.

2. **Increased Effectiveness:** Proper posture ensures that muscles engage optimally, enhancing the effectiveness of exercises and leading to better results.

3. **Enhanced Body Awareness:** Regular practice of aligning the body correctly promotes a heightened sense of body awareness, both during workouts and in daily activities.

4. **Improved Postural Habits:** By reinforcing proper alignment principles in Wall Pilates, individuals can carry these habits into their everyday lives, leading to better posture and reduced discomfort.

Breathing Techniques

Comprehensive Overview of Breathing Techniques in Wall Pilates

Importance of Breath in Wall Pilates:

1. **Core Engagement:** Breath acts as a catalyst for core activation in Wall Pilates. Proper breathing patterns facilitate the engagement of deep abdominal muscles, enhancing stability and control during exercises against the wall.

2. **Mind-Body Connection:** Conscious breathing fosters a strong mind-body connection. It allows practitioners to synchronize movement with breath, promoting fluidity and efficiency in exercises.

3. **Energy and Relaxation:** Utilizing breath effectively aids in conserving energy and reducing tension. It can be both energizing and relaxing, depending on the emphasis placed on different breathing patterns.

Basic Breathing Patterns in Wall Pilates:

1. **Lateral Thoracic Breathing:** This involves inhaling laterally into the ribcage, expanding the ribcage sideways, and exhaling to draw the ribs back in. It encourages three-dimensional breathing, facilitating better movement and expansion in the torso.

2. **Diaphragmatic Breathing:** Emphasizing the use of the diaphragm, this technique involves inhaling deeply into the lower abdomen, allowing it to expand, and exhaling to release the breath fully. It encourages relaxation and full oxygenation of the body.

Integration of Breath with Movement:

1. **Inhalation and Exhalation Phases:** Wall Pilates often incorporates specific breathing patterns tied to movements. For example, inhaling during preparatory or expansive movements and exhaling during the exertion or contracting phase.

2. **Pacing and Rhythm:** Establishing a rhythm between breath and movement fosters a smooth flow during exercises against the wall. Coordinating inhalations and exhalations with specific movements enhances control and precision.

Techniques to Enhance Breathing in Wall Pilates:

1. **Mindful Awareness:** Bringing attention to the breath is fundamental. Practitioners are encouraged to focus on the quality and depth of their breath, ensuring it remains steady and controlled throughout the workout.

2. **Cueing and Visualization:** Instructors use verbal cues to guide participants in synchronizing their breath with movements against the wall. Visualization techniques, such as imagining the breath reaching specific areas of the body, aid in deepening the breath experience.

Benefits of Incorporating Proper Breathing Techniques:

1. **Enhanced Core Activation:** Proper breathing facilitates better engagement of core muscles, enhancing stability and control during Wall Pilates exercises.

2. **Improved Focus and Concentration:** Conscious breathing promotes mindfulness, aiding in focus and concentration during workouts, leading to better performance.

3. **Reduced Tension and Stress:** Utilizing breath as a tool for relaxation helps in reducing muscular tension and stress, promoting a sense of calmness and well-being.

4. **Efficient Oxygenation:** Effective breathing ensures optimal oxygenation of muscles, enhancing endurance and reducing fatigue during workouts.

5. **Mind-Body Coordination:** Synchronizing breath with movement fosters a harmonious connection between the body and mind, promoting efficient and controlled movements against the wall.

Core Engagement

Understanding the Core:

1. **Anatomy of the Core:** The core is not limited to just the abdominal muscles but encompasses a complex group of muscles, including the deep stabilizing muscles of the abdomen, back, pelvis, and even the diaphragm and pelvic floor.

2. **Functional Role of the Core:** The core serves as the body's center of support and stabilization. In Wall Pilates, activating and engaging these muscles is vital for maintaining proper alignment, control, and balance.

Principles of Core Engagement in Wall Pilates:

1. **Initiation and Control:** Core engagement begins with awareness and intentional activation of these muscles. Initiating movements from a stable core ensures controlled and efficient execution of exercises against the wall.

2. **Integrated Movement:** Wall Pilates emphasizes integrating core engagement into all movements. This includes both static poses against the wall and dynamic exercises, ensuring that the core muscles remain active and supportive throughout.

Techniques for Effective Core Engagement:

1. **Breath and Core Activation:** Breath plays a crucial role in initiating and supporting core engagement. Coordinating breath with movements against the wall aids in deepening core activation and stability.

2. **Mindful Focus:** Practitioners are encouraged to maintain continuous awareness of their core muscles. Focusing on these muscles during exercises ensures they remain engaged, supporting posture and movement.

Key Elements of Core Engagement in Different Wall Pilates Exercises:

1. **Static Wall Poses:** Maintaining static positions against the wall, such as wall squats or wall planks, relies heavily on sustained core engagement for stability and support.

2. **Dynamic Movements:** Dynamic exercises like wall roll-downs or wall push-ups require continuous core activation to control movement and maintain proper form against the wall.

Progressions and Variations to Enhance Core Engagement:

1. **Increasing Challenge:** Progressing from simpler to more complex exercises gradually challenges the core muscles further, enhancing their strength and endurance in Wall Pilates.

2. **Variations in Resistance:** Incorporating props or altering body positioning against the wall can intensify core engagement. For instance, using resistance bands or instability tools can add a new dimension to core-focused exercises.

Benefits of Effective Core Engagement in Wall Pilates:

1. **Enhanced Stability and Control:** Activating the core muscles ensures better stability, control, and balance during exercises against the wall, minimizing the risk of injury.

2. **Improved Posture:** A strong core supports proper spinal alignment, leading to better posture both during workouts and in daily activities.

3. **Increased Strength and Endurance:** Regular engagement of the core muscles in Wall Pilates leads to improved strength and endurance, benefiting overall physical fitness.

4. **Injury Prevention:** A well-engaged core acts as a protective mechanism, reducing the strain on other muscles and joints and preventing potential injuries.

5. **Functional Movement:** Strong core muscles facilitate better functional movement patterns, enhancing performance in various activities beyond the workout setting.

Wall Basics

Using the Wall for Support

Introduction to Wall Support:

1. **Purpose of Wall Support:** In Wall Pilates, the wall serves as a stabilizing element, providing support and assistance during exercises. It aids practitioners in maintaining proper alignment, balance, and controlled movements.

2. **Safety and Stability:** Utilizing the wall for support offers a secure environment for individuals, especially beginners or those with limited mobility, to perform exercises with reduced risk of injury.

Principles of Using the Wall for Support:

1. **Alignment and Contact Points:** Understanding how to position the body against the wall is crucial. Emphasizing alignment of specific body parts, such as the back, shoulders, or feet, against the wall ensures optimal support and engagement of targeted muscles.

2. **Controlled Engagement:** The wall acts as a point of contact for controlled engagement of muscles. It allows individuals to focus on specific muscle groups while performing movements, promoting proper form and stability.

Various Uses of the Wall for Support:

1. **Stabilizing Poses:** Wall Pilates includes static poses where the wall provides stability, such as wall squats, wall sits, or leaning exercises, allowing individuals to focus on alignment and muscle engagement.

2. **Assisted Movements:** The wall can assist in performing certain exercises that might be challenging initially. For example, using the wall for balance during leg raises or providing support during stretches.

Techniques and Tips for Optimal Wall Support:

1. **Body Awareness:** Practitioners are guided to develop a keen sense of body awareness against the wall, ensuring proper alignment and engagement of muscles.

2. **Progressive Use of Wall Support:** Beginning with basic exercises against the wall and gradually progressing to more complex movements ensures a gradual adaptation to utilizing the wall for support.

Benefits of Utilizing the Wall for Support:

1. **Enhanced Stability and Control:** The wall offers a stable foundation, enabling individuals to focus on proper technique and control during exercises, leading to enhanced stability.

2. **Improved Alignment:** Using the wall as a guide helps in maintaining correct alignment, promoting better posture and reducing strain on muscles and joints.

3. **Accessible for All Levels:** The wall serves as a versatile tool, making Wall Pilates accessible to individuals of varying fitness levels and abilities, allowing for modifications and adaptations.

Integration into Wall Pilates Workouts:

1. **Incorporating Wall Support into Exercises:** The section explores how practitioners can seamlessly integrate the wall for support into different exercises and workout routines for a comprehensive Pilates practice.

2. **Customization and Adaptation:** Understanding how to adapt exercises using the wall for support allows individuals to customize workouts according to their needs and goals.

Safety Measures and Precautions

Importance of Safety in Wall Pilates:

1. **Injury Prevention:** Safety measures aim to minimize the risk of injury during Wall Pilates exercises, ensuring a safe and comfortable experience for practitioners.

2. **Foundational Understanding:** Emphasizing safety measures provides practitioners with foundational knowledge on how to approach exercises against the wall, fostering a secure environment for practice.

Key Safety Measures and Precautions:

1. **Proper Warm-Up:** Beginning with a comprehensive warm-up routine prepares the body for exercises, increasing blood flow to muscles and reducing the risk of strains or injuries.

2. **Progression and Gradual Adaptation:** Gradually progressing from simpler to more challenging exercises allows the body to adapt, reducing the likelihood of overexertion or strain.

3. **Correct Alignment and Form:** Stressing the importance of maintaining proper alignment and form against the wall prevents unnecessary stress on muscles and joints, reducing the risk of injury.

4. **Breath Awareness:** Educating practitioners on the significance of coordinating breath with movements promotes control and reduces the risk of breath-holding or improper breathing techniques that can lead to strain.

Safety Guidelines During Wall Pilates Workouts:

1. **Instruction and Supervision:** Recommending practicing under the guidance of a certified instructor ensures proper technique and form, especially for beginners or those unfamiliar with Wall Pilates.

2. **Respecting Individual Limits:** Encouraging practitioners to listen to their bodies and respect their limits during exercises, avoiding overexertion or pushing beyond their comfort zones.

3. **Proper Equipment and Environment:** Ensuring the use of suitable equipment and a safe environment for Wall Pilates workouts minimizes the risk of accidents or injuries.

Addressing Preexisting Conditions or Injuries:

1. **Consultation with Healthcare Professionals:** Advising individuals with preexisting health conditions or injuries to seek advice from healthcare professionals before engaging in Wall Pilates ensures exercise suitability and safety.
2. **Modifications and Adaptations:** Offering modifications or alternative exercises for individuals with specific health concerns allows them to participate safely and effectively.

Emphasizing Continuous Awareness:

1. **Body Awareness:** Encouraging practitioners to maintain continuous awareness of their bodies during exercises helps in identifying discomfort or strain, allowing for timely adjustments.
2. **Mindful Practice:** Promoting a mindful approach to Wall Pilates cultivates an environment where practitioners prioritize their safety and well-being throughout the workout.

Chapter 2: Wall Pilates Exercises

1. Wall Squats Variations

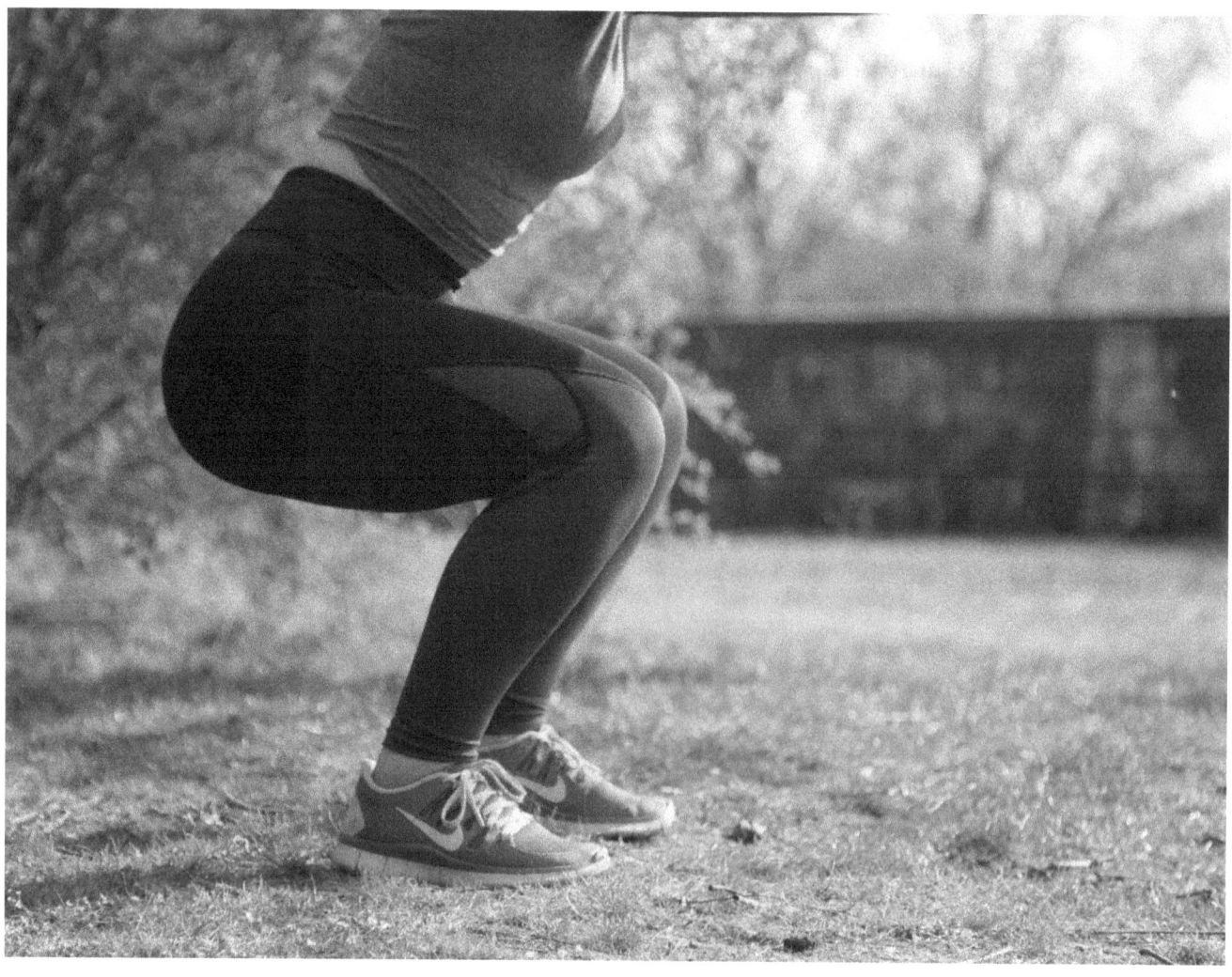

1. Basic Wall Squats

Description:

The foundational Wall Squat involves leaning against the wall, feet hip-width apart, and sliding down until the thighs are parallel to the floor. It emphasizes proper alignment and engages major lower body muscles.

Technique:

1. Stand against the wall with the feet about hip-width apart and slightly away from the wall.
2. Lower the body by sliding down the wall, keeping the back straight and the knees aligned with the ankles.
3. Hold the squat position for a few seconds, ensuring the thighs are parallel to the floor.
4. Push through the heels to return to the starting position.

Benefits:

- Strengthens quadriceps, hamstrings, and glutes.
- Emphasizes proper squatting form and alignment.

2. Wall Squats with Leg Raises

Description:

This variation adds complexity by incorporating leg raises, challenging stability and balance while engaging core muscles and hip flexors.

Technique:

1. Perform a basic wall squat.

2. Lift one leg straight out in front, keeping it parallel to the floor.
3. Lower the leg back down and repeat on the other side.

Benefits:

- Enhances balance and stability.
- Engages core and hip flexor muscles for added strength.

3. Wall Squats with Ball Squeeze

Description:

Utilizes a small ball between the knees during wall squats, adding resistance and engaging inner thigh muscles.

Technique:

1. Place a small ball between the knees while performing a basic wall squat.
2. Squeeze the ball gently throughout the squat movement, engaging the inner thighs.

Benefits:

- Targets inner thigh muscles (adductors) for increased strength.
- Adds resistance to the squat movement.

4. Wall Squats with Arm Raises

Description:

Incorporates arm movements to engage upper body muscles while maintaining the lower body squat position against the wall.

Technique:

1. Perform a basic wall squat.
2. While in the squat position, raise the arms overhead, keeping them straight.
3. Lower the arms back down and repeat.

Benefits:

- Engages shoulder, chest, and upper back muscles.
- Increases overall body coordination.

5. One-Legged Wall Squats

Description:

A challenging variation that focuses on single-leg strength and stability, requiring more control and balance.

Technique:

1. Stand on one leg away from the wall.
2. Perform a squat motion on the standing leg, using the wall for support if needed.
3. Maintain control and balance while lowering and raising the body.

Benefits:

- Enhances single-leg strength and balance.
- Targets stabilizing muscles throughout the body.

6. Wall Squats with Resistance Band

Description:

Incorporates a resistance band around the thighs to add resistance and intensity to the wall squat movement.

Technique:

1. Place a resistance band just above the knees.
2. Perform a basic wall squat, pressing against the resistance of the band throughout the movement.

Benefits:

- Intensifies the squat movement by adding resistance.
- Engages outer thigh and hip muscles.

7. Dynamic Wall Squats

Description:

Adds a dynamic element to the wall squat by incorporating a pulsing or bouncing movement, increasing time under tension.

Technique:

1. Perform a basic wall squat.
2. Add a small bouncing or pulsing movement within the squat position, maintaining control and stability.

Benefits:

- Increases muscular endurance and strength.
- Enhances stability through controlled movement.

8. Wall Squats with Calf Raises

Description:

Combines the squat motion with calf raises, targeting the calves and adding a dynamic element to the exercise.

Technique:

1. Perform a basic wall squat.
2. From the squat position, rise onto the balls of the feet to perform a calf raise.
3. Lower back into the squat position and repeat the movement.

Benefits:

- Engages calf muscles for strength and stability.
- Adds an extra challenge to the lower body workout.

9. Wall Squats with Rotation

Description:

Incorporates rotational movements to engage core muscles and add a twist to the traditional wall squat.

Technique:

1. Perform a basic wall squat.

2. While in the squat position, rotate the torso to one side, then return to the center and rotate to the other side, alternating rotations.

Benefits:

- Engages oblique and core muscles.
- Enhances mobility and flexibility through rotational movement.

10. Wall Squat Holds with Arm Variations

Description:

Focuses on isometric holds with variations in arm positions, intensifying the challenge and engaging different upper body muscles.

Technique:

1. Perform a basic wall squat and hold the position.
2. Experiment with various arm positions, such as extended overhead, crossed in front of the chest, or at shoulder height, while maintaining the squat.

Benefits:

- Targets different upper body muscles (shoulders, chest, arms) while holding the squat position.
- Increases endurance and challenges stability.

2. Wall Roll-Down Variations

1. Controlled Roll-Downs

Description:

A foundational Wall Roll-Down exercise focusing on controlled spinal movement and flexibility.

Technique:

1. Stand with your back against the wall, feet hip-width apart.
2. Inhale, lengthening through the spine.
3. Exhale, sequentially rolling down through the spine, vertebra by vertebra, until reaching a comfortable forward fold.
4. Inhale to maintain the position, then exhale as you roll back up to standing, stacking each vertebra.

Benefits:

- Improves spinal mobility and flexibility.
- Engages core muscles for controlled movement.

2. Roll-Downs with Arm Movements

Description:

Incorporates arm movements to enhance shoulder mobility and upper body engagement during the roll-down.

Addison Mitchell

Technique:

1. Perform controlled roll-downs against the wall.
2. At the bottom of the roll-down, reach the arms overhead or out to the sides.
3. Keep the arms in position as you roll back up, maintaining control and engagement.

Benefits:

- Increases shoulder mobility and flexibility.
- Engages upper body muscles for a full-body movement.

3. Wall Roll-Downs for Flexibility

Description:

Focuses on maximizing the stretch and flexibility through a deeper roll-down motion.

Technique:

1. Start with controlled roll-downs, aiming for a deeper forward fold.
2. Once at the bottom of the movement, reach towards the floor or try to touch the toes to deepen the stretch.
3. Roll back up slowly, feeling the lengthening of the spine.

Benefits:

- Enhances hamstring and back flexibility.
- Promotes a deeper stretch through the entire spine.

4. Roll-Downs with Spinal Twist

Description:

Introduces a rotational movement to the roll-down exercise, targeting spinal mobility and core engagement.

Technique:

1. Perform controlled roll-downs against the wall.
2. At the bottom of the movement, rotate the torso to one side, feeling the stretch through the spine.
3. Return to center and roll back up, alternating sides for the twist.

Benefits:

- Increases spinal mobility and rotation.
- Engages core muscles for stabilization.

5. Wall Roll-Downs with Resistance Band

Description:

Incorporates a resistance band to add challenge and intensity to the roll-down movement.

Technique:

1. Place a resistance band around the feet or thighs.
2. Perform controlled roll-downs, maintaining tension in the resistance band throughout the movement.
3. Roll back up, focusing on controlled resistance against the band.

Benefits:

- Increases resistance for added muscle engagement.
- Challenges stability and control throughout the movement.

6. Wall Roll-Downs with Pelvic Tilt

Description:

Combines pelvic tilts with the roll-down motion to engage lower abdominal muscles and improve pelvic mobility.

Technique:

1. Perform controlled roll-downs against the wall.
2. At the bottom of the movement, engage the lower abdominals and tilt the pelvis forward and backward.
3. Roll back up, maintaining control and pelvic engagement.

Benefits:

- Targets lower abdominal muscles and pelvic mobility.
- Enhances control and coordination in pelvic movements.

7. Wall Roll-Downs with Leg Slide

Description:

Adds a leg sliding movement to the roll-down to engage hamstring muscles and improve lower body flexibility.

Technique:

1. Perform controlled roll-downs against the wall.
2. At the bottom of the movement, slide one leg straight out in front while maintaining the forward fold.
3. Return the leg and roll back up, alternating legs for each repetition.

Benefits:
- Increases hamstring flexibility and mobility.
- Engages leg muscles for a deeper stretch.

8. Dynamic Wall Roll-Downs

Description:

Incorporates a dynamic bouncing or pulsing movement within the roll-down exercise to increase time under tension.

Technique:
1. Perform controlled roll-downs against the wall.
2. Add a small bouncing or pulsing movement while in the forward fold, maintaining control and engagement.
3. Roll back up, focusing on the controlled movement.

Benefits:
- Enhances muscle endurance and strength.
- Increases time under tension for deeper engagement.

9. Wall Roll-Downs with Arm Circles

Description:

Introduces circular arm movements to engage shoulder muscles and increase upper body mobility.

Technique:

1. Perform controlled roll-downs against the wall.
2. At the bottom of the movement, circle the arms forward or backward, maintaining the forward fold.
3. Return the arms to the sides and roll back up, maintaining control.

Benefits:

- Improves shoulder mobility and flexibility.
- Engages upper body muscles for a full-body movement.

10. Wall Roll-Downs with Ball Squeeze

Description:

Incorporates a ball squeeze between the knees to add resistance and engage inner thigh muscles during the roll-down movement.

Technique:

1. Place a small ball between the knees.
2. Perform controlled roll-downs against the wall, maintaining the ball squeeze throughout the movement.

3. Roll back up, focusing on controlled resistance against the ball.

Benefits:

- Targets inner thigh muscles for added strength.
- Adds resistance for increased muscle engagement.

3. Wall Push-Ups Variations

1. Basic Wall Push-Ups

Description:

The foundational Wall Push-Up involves using the wall for support while performing a push-up motion, targeting chest, arms, and shoulder muscles.

Technique:

1. Stand facing the wall at arm's length, place palms on the wall at shoulder height.
2. Lean forward, bending elbows to lower the chest toward the wall.
3. Push back to the starting position without locking elbows.

Benefits:

- Engages chest, triceps, and shoulders.
- Suitable for beginners to build upper body strength.

2. Decline Wall Push-Ups

Description:

Increases intensity by elevating the feet, challenging upper body strength and stability.

Technique:

1. Place hands on the wall and step back, elevating the feet on a sturdy platform.

2. Perform a push-up motion by lowering the chest toward the wall and pushing back up.

Benefits:
- Intensifies the exercise for increased upper body strength.
- Engages core muscles for stability.

3. Incline Wall Push-Ups

Description:

Reduces intensity by positioning the hands higher on the wall, suitable for individuals with limited upper body strength.

Technique:
1. Stand facing the wall and place hands higher than shoulder height.
2. Lean forward, bending elbows to perform a push-up motion against the wall.

Benefits:
- Allows individuals to perform push-ups with reduced upper body strain.
- Targets chest and shoulder muscles effectively.

4. One-Arm Wall Push-Ups

Description:

Focuses on unilateral strength by performing push-ups with one arm, challenging stability and balance.

Technique:

1. Place one hand on the wall and slightly stagger the feet for balance.
2. Lower the chest toward the wall, keeping the body straight, and push back up.

Benefits:

- Enhances unilateral upper body strength.
- Engages core muscles for stability.

5. Wall Push-Ups with Shoulder Taps

Description:

Adds a dynamic element by incorporating shoulder taps during the push-up, targeting shoulder stability and core engagement.

Technique:

1. Perform a standard wall push-up.
2. At the top of the push-up, tap one hand to the opposite shoulder while maintaining stability.

Benefits:

- Engages shoulder stabilizers and core muscles.
- Enhances coordination and balance.

6. Wall Push-Ups with Leg Raises

Description:

Introduces leg raises to engage lower body muscles while performing wall push-ups.

Technique:

1. Perform a standard wall push-up.
2. At the top of the push-up, lift one leg off the ground, keeping it straight, and return to the floor.

Benefits:

- Engages lower body muscles for added strength.
- Challenges stability and balance.

7. Plyometric Wall Push-Ups

Description:

Incorporates a explosive movement into the push-up, increasing power and strength.

Technique:

1. Perform a standard wall push-up.
2. Push away from the wall explosively, allowing the hands to leave the wall before catching the body.

Benefits:

- Builds explosive upper body strength.
- Increases power and muscle recruitment.

8. Wall Push-Ups with Resistance Band

Description:

Utilizes a resistance band to increase resistance and intensify the push-up movement.

Technique:

1. Place a resistance band around the back and hold the ends with each hand.
2. Perform a standard wall push-up while maintaining tension in the band.

Benefits:

- Adds resistance for increased muscle engagement.
- Challenges upper body strength.

9. Diamond Wall Push-Ups

Description:

Positions the hands closer together in a diamond shape to target triceps and chest muscles.

Technique:

1. Place hands on the wall close together, forming a diamond shape with thumbs and index fingers.
2. Perform a standard wall push-up with elbows close to the body.

Benefits:

- Targets triceps and inner chest muscles.
- Challenges upper body strength in a different way.

10. Wall Push-Up Holds

Description:

Focuses on isometric contraction by holding the push-up position against the wall.

Technique:

1. Perform a standard wall push-up and hold the lowered position with elbows bent.
2. Maintain the hold for a specific duration before pushing back to the starting position.

Benefits:

- Builds endurance in chest, shoulder, and triceps muscles.
- Increases time under tension for muscle engagement.

4. Wall Angels Variations

1. Basic Wall Angels

Description:

The foundational Wall Angel exercise involves performing arm movements against the wall to improve shoulder mobility and posture.

Technique:

1. Stand with the back against the wall, arms by the sides.
2. Slowly raise arms, keeping them in contact with the wall, until they form a "Y" shape overhead.
3. Return arms to the starting position while maintaining contact with the wall.

Benefits:

- Improves shoulder mobility and flexibility.
- Helps in correcting posture.

2. Wall Angel Holds

Description:

Focuses on isometric holds at different points in the Wall Angel movement to increase time under tension.

Technique:

1. Perform a basic Wall Angel by raising arms against the wall.
2. Hold the arms at various angles (e.g., 45 degrees, 90 degrees) for a specific duration before returning to the starting position.

Benefits:

- Increases muscular endurance in shoulder muscles.
- Enhances control and stability in different arm positions.

3. Dynamic Wall Angels

Description:

Incorporates a dynamic element by adding small pulses or movements during the Wall Angel exercise.

Technique:

1. Perform a basic Wall Angel.
2. Add small pulses or movements (upward or downward) while maintaining contact with the wall.

Benefits:

- Increases time under tension for muscle engagement.
- Improves shoulder joint mobility.

4. Wall Angels with Resistance Band

Description:

Utilizes a resistance band to add challenge and intensity to the Wall Angel movement.

Technique:

1. Hold a resistance band in both hands, positioned against the wall.
2. Perform the Wall Angel movement while maintaining tension in the resistance band.

Benefits:

- Adds resistance for increased muscle engagement.
- Strengthens shoulder muscles.

5. One-Arm Wall Angels

Description:

Focuses on unilateral shoulder movement by performing the Wall Angel exercise with one arm at a time.

Technique:

1. Position one arm against the wall and perform the Wall Angel movement with that arm.
2. Repeat the movement with the opposite arm.

Benefits:

- Enhances unilateral shoulder mobility and control.
- Helps in identifying and addressing asymmetry in shoulder movement.

6. Wall Angel Circles

Description:

Incorporates circular arm movements during the Wall Angel exercise to increase shoulder joint mobility.

Technique:

1. Perform a basic Wall Angel.
2. Add circular movements with arms while maintaining contact with the wall.

Benefits:

- Increases shoulder joint range of motion.
- Enhances shoulder flexibility and mobility.

7. Wall Angel Pulses

Description:

Focuses on small, controlled pulses at various points in the Wall Angel movement to challenge shoulder muscles.

Technique:

1. Perform a basic Wall Angel.
2. Add small pulses or movements at different angles while maintaining contact with the wall.

Benefits:

- Increases muscle activation and endurance in the shoulders.
- Helps in refining control and precision in arm movements.

8. Wall Angel Twist

Description:

Introduces a rotational element to the Wall Angel movement to enhance thoracic spine mobility.

Technique:

1. Perform a basic Wall Angel.
2. Add a gentle twist through the torso while maintaining arm contact with the wall.

Benefits:

- Increases thoracic spine mobility.
- Engages core muscles for stability.

9. Wall Angels with Leg Movements

Description:

Incorporates leg movements to engage lower body muscles while performing Wall Angels.

Technique:

1. Perform a basic Wall Angel.
2. Add leg movements (e.g., marching in place, lifting knees) while maintaining arm contact with the wall.

Benefits:

- Engages lower body muscles for added stability and balance.

- Increases overall body coordination.

10. Wall Angel Flow

Description:

Combines various Wall Angel variations into a seamless flow of movements for a comprehensive workout.

Technique:

1. Sequence different Wall Angel variations (e.g., holds, pulses, circles) into a continuous flow of movements.
2. Perform the flow of Wall Angel variations with controlled and fluid transitions.

Benefits:

- Works on different aspects of shoulder mobility and strength.
- Provides a comprehensive workout for the shoulders and upper body.

5. Wall Plank Variations

1. Basic Wall Plank

Description:

The foundational Wall Plank involves assuming a plank position against the wall, engaging core and upper body muscles for stability.

Technique:

1. Stand facing the wall, place hands on the wall at shoulder height.
2. Walk feet back until body forms a straight line from head to heels.
3. Engage core muscles and hold the position, maintaining a neutral spine.

Benefits:

- Engages core, shoulder, and arm muscles.
- Builds upper body and core strength.

2. Wall Plank Holds with Arm Variations

Description:

Introduces variations in arm positions to engage different upper body muscles during the wall plank hold.

Technique:

1. Assume the basic wall plank position.

2. Experiment with different arm variations: extended overhead, crossed in front, at shoulder height, etc., while maintaining the plank.

Benefits:

- Engages various upper body muscles for stability.
- Increases endurance in different arm positions.

3. One-Legged Wall Plank

Description:

Challenges stability and balance by lifting one leg off the ground during the wall plank hold.

Technique:

1. Assume the basic wall plank position.
2. Lift one leg off the ground, keeping it straight, and hold the position without compromising the plank posture.

Benefits:

- Engages core muscles and improves balance.
- Increases unilateral leg strength.

4. Wall Plank with Leg Lifts

Description:

Incorporates leg lifts to engage lower body muscles while maintaining the wall plank position.

Technique:

1. Assume the basic wall plank position.
2. Lift one leg off the ground, keeping it straight, and perform small leg lifts while holding the plank.

Benefits:

- Engages lower body muscles for added strength.
- Challenges stability and balance.

5. Wall Plank Twists

Description:

Introduces a rotational element by twisting the torso during the wall plank hold, engaging core and oblique muscles.

Technique:

1. Assume the basic wall plank position.
2. Rotate the torso to one side, bringing the arm towards the opposite hip, then return to the plank position and alternate sides.

Benefits:

- Engages oblique and core muscles for rotational stability.
- Increases thoracic spine mobility.

6. Wall Plank with Knee Tucks

Description:

Adds a dynamic element by performing knee tucks during the wall plank, engaging core and hip flexor muscles.

Technique:

1. Assume the basic wall plank position.
2. Alternate bringing each knee towards the chest while maintaining the plank posture.

Benefits:

- Engages core and hip flexor muscles for strength.
- Increases mobility and flexibility in the hips.

7. Wall Plank Shoulder Taps

Description:

Incorporates shoulder taps to challenge stability and core engagement during the wall plank hold.

Technique:

1. Assume the basic wall plank position.
2. Lift one hand and tap the opposite shoulder, then alternate sides while maintaining a stable plank.

Benefits:

- Engages core muscles for stability.
- Improves coordination and balance.

8. Wall Plank with Arm Reaches

Description:

Adds a reaching movement with arms to engage shoulder and upper back muscles during the wall plank.

Technique:

1. Assume the basic wall plank position.
2. Reach one arm straight out in front, then return to the plank and alternate sides.

Benefits:

- Engages shoulder and upper back muscles.
- Increases shoulder mobility and flexibility.

9. Wall Plank with Side Leg Raises

Description:

Targets outer hip muscles by incorporating side leg raises during the wall plank.

Technique:

1. Assume the basic wall plank position.
2. Lift one leg out to the side while maintaining the plank, then return to the center and alternate sides.

Benefits:

- Engages outer hip muscles for added strength.
- Challenges stability and balance.

10. Wall Plank Flow

Description:

Combines various wall plank variations into a continuous flow of movements for a comprehensive workout.

Technique:

1. Sequence different wall plank variations (e.g., leg lifts, twists, arm reaches) into a continuous flow of movements.
2. Perform the flow of wall plank variations with controlled and fluid transitions.

Benefits:

- Works on different aspects of core and upper body strength.
- Provides a comprehensive workout for the entire body.

Chapter 3: Advanced Wall Pilates Workouts

Challenging Wall Pilates Sequences

1. Wall Pilates Full-Body Flow Sequence

Warm-Up:

- **Arm Circles:** 1 minute forward, 1 minute backward.
- **Leg Swings:** 1 minute each leg.

Sequence:

1. **Wall Squats with Arm Raises:** 15 reps.
2. **Wall Plank Hold:** 30 seconds.
3. **Wall Angels with Resistance Band:** 12 reps.
4. **Wall Push-Ups with Rotation:** 10 reps each side.
5. **Wall Plank Shoulder Taps:** 20 taps (10 each side).
6. **Wall Roll-Downs with Leg Slide:** 10 reps.
7. **One-Legged Wall Plank Hold:** 20 seconds each leg.
8. **Wall Squat Leg Raises:** 12 reps each leg.
9. **Wall Plank with Knee Tucks:** 12 tucks each side.
10. **Dynamic Wall Angels:** 10 reps with small pulses.

Cool Down:

- **Child's Pose:** 1 minute.
- **Standing Forward Fold:** 1 minute.

2. Advanced Wall Pilates Strength Circuit

Warm-Up:

- **High Knees:** 1 minute.
- **Arm Reaches:** 30 seconds each side.

Circuit (Repeat 3 times):

1. **Decline Wall Push-Ups:** 12 reps.
2. **Wall Squats with Ball Squeeze:** 15 reps.
3. **Wall Plank Leg Lifts:** 10 lifts each leg.
4. **One-Legged Wall Plank with Arm Variations:** 20 seconds each leg.
5. **Wall Angels with Leg Raises:** 10 reps.
6. **Wall Plank Flow:** 1 round integrating 5 variations.

Cool Down:

- **Seated Spinal Twist:** 1 minute each side.
- **Deep Breathing Exercise:** 2 minutes focusing on slow, controlled breaths.

3. Wall Pilates Dynamic Power Sequence

Warm-Up:

- **Standing Marches:** 1 minute.
- **Arm Circles:** 1 minute forward, 1 minute backward.

Sequence:

1. **Plyometric Wall Push-Ups:** 15 reps.
2. **Wall Plank with Knee to Elbow:** 12 reps each side.
3. **Wall Squats with Leg Raises and Calf Raises:** 10 reps.
4. **Wall Plank Flow with Arm Reaches and Twists:** 2 rounds.
5. **Wall Angels with Dynamic Pulses:** 15 reps.
6. **Wall Squat Leg Raises with Arm Circles:** 12 reps each leg.
7. **One-Legged Wall Plank with Leg Lifts:** 10 lifts each leg.
8. **Wall Roll-Downs with Arm Circles:** 10 reps.

Cool Down:

- **Seated Forward Fold:** 1 minute.
- **Shoulder Stretch against Wall:** 30 seconds each arm.

4. Wall Pilates Core and Stability Fusion

Warm-Up:
- **Leg Swings:** 1 minute each leg.
- **Arm Circles:** 30 seconds forward, 30 seconds backward.

Fusion (Repeat 3 times):
1. **Wall Plank with Knee Tucks and Arm Reaches:** 10 reps each side.
2. **Wall Squats with Leg Raises and Arm Circles:** 12 reps.
3. **Wall Plank with Shoulder Taps and Leg Lifts:** 10 taps and lifts each side.
4. **Dynamic Wall Angels with Resistance Band:** 15 reps.
5. **Wall Push-Ups with Decline and Rotation:** 10 reps each side.
6. **One-Legged Wall Plank with Dynamic Arm Variations:** 20 seconds each leg.

Cool Down:
- **Seated Spinal Twist:** 1 minute each side.
- **Deep Breathing Exercise:** 2 minutes focusing on slow, controlled breaths.

5. Wall Pilates Advanced Flexibility Sequence

Warm-Up:

- **High Knees:** 1 minute.
- **Arm Reaches:** 30 seconds each side.

Sequence:

1. **Wall Squats with Forward Fold:** 10 reps.
2. **Wall Plank Hold with Leg Pulls:** 20 seconds each leg.
3. **Wall Roll-Downs with Leg Slide and Toe Touches:** 10 reps.
4. **Wall Angels with Full Range Arm Circles:** 12 reps.
5. **Wall Plank with Pike Position:** 10 reps.
6. **Dynamic Wall Squats with Arm Swings:** 15 reps.
7. **Wall Push-Ups with Chest Stretch:** 12 reps.
8. **One-Legged Wall Plank with Side Stretch:** 15 seconds each leg.

Cool Down:

- **Seated Forward Fold:** 1 minute.
- **Shoulder Stretch against Wall:** 30 seconds each arm.

6. Wall Pilates Strength and Endurance Fusion

Warm-Up:

- **Standing Marches:** 1 minute.
- **Arm Circles:** 1 minute forward, 1 minute backward.

Fusion (Repeat 3 times):

1. **Decline Wall Push-Ups:** 15 reps.
2. **Wall Plank Holds with Arm Variations:** 30 seconds each variation.
3. **Wall Squats with Ball Squeeze and Arm Raises:** 12 reps.
4. **Wall Plank Leg Lifts with Knee Tucks:** 10 reps each side.
5. **One-Legged Wall Plank with Dynamic Arm Movements:** 20 seconds each leg.
6. **Wall Angels with Resistance Band and Pulses:** 15 reps.

Cool Down:

- **Child's Pose:** 1 minute.
- **Standing Forward Fold:** 1 minute.

7. Dynamic Wall Pilates Core Challenge

Warm-Up:

- **Leg Swings:** 1 minute each leg.
- **Arm Circles:** 30 seconds forward, 30 seconds backward.

Core Challenge (Repeat 3 times):

1. **Wall Plank with Knee to Elbow and Leg Lifts:** 10 reps each side.
2. **Wall Squats with Leg Raises and Arm Reaches:** 12 reps.
3. **Wall Plank Shoulder Taps with Side Leg Raises:** 10 taps and lifts each side.
4. **Dynamic Wall Angels with Full Range Pulses:** 15 reps.
5. **Wall Push-Ups with Decline and Rotation:** 12 reps each side.
6. **One-Legged Wall Plank with Dynamic Arm Circles:** 20 seconds each leg.

Cool Down:

- **Seated Spinal Twist:** 1 minute each side.
- **Deep Breathing Exercise:** 2 minutes focusing on slow, controlled breaths.

8. Wall Pilates Functional Strength Circuit

Warm-Up:

- **High Knees:** 1 minute.
- **Arm Reaches:** 30 seconds each side.

Circuit (Repeat 3 times):

1. **Wall Squats with Leg Raises and Calf Raises:** 15 reps.
2. **Wall Plank Flow with Knee Tucks and Arm Reaches:** 1 round.
3. **Plyometric Wall Push-Ups:** 12 reps.
4. **Wall Angels with Resistance Band:** 15 reps.
5. **One-Legged Wall Squats with Arm Circles:** 12 reps each leg.
6. **Wall Plank with Shoulder Taps and Leg Lifts:** 10 taps and lifts each side.

Cool Down:

- **Seated Forward Fold:** 1 minute.
- **Shoulder Stretch against Wall:** 30 seconds each arm.

9. Wall Pilates Mobility and Flexibility Sequence

Warm-Up:

- **Standing Marches:** 1 minute.
- **Arm Circles:** 1 minute forward, 1 minute backward.

Sequence:

1. **Wall Squats with Forward Fold and Toe Touches:** 12 reps.
2. **Wall Plank Hold with Leg Swings:** 15 swings each leg.
3. **Wall Roll-Downs with Arm Circles and Side Bends:** 10 reps.
4. **Wall Angels with Full Range Dynamic Pulses:** 12 reps.
5. **Wall Plank with Pike Position and Hip Flexor Stretch:** 10 reps.
6. **Dynamic Wall Squats with Arm Swings and Twist:** 15 reps.
7. **Wall Push-Ups with Chest Stretch and Rotation:** 12 reps.
8. **One-Legged Wall Plank with Side Stretch and Reach:** 15 seconds each leg.

Cool Down:

- **Seated Forward Fold:** 1 minute.
- **Shoulder Stretch against Wall:** 30 seconds each arm.

10. Wall Pilates Dynamic Power and Strength Circuit

Warm-Up:

- **High Knees:** 1 minute.
- **Arm Reaches:** 30 seconds each side.

Circuit (Repeat 3 times):

1. **Plyometric Wall Push-Ups:** 15 reps.
2. **Wall Plank with Knee to Elbow and Leg Lifts:** 12 reps each side.
3. **Wall Squats with Leg Raises and Arm Circles:** 12 reps.
4. **Wall Plank Flow with Arm Reaches and Twists:** 2 rounds.
5. **Wall Angels with Dynamic Pulses:** 15 reps.
6. **Wall Squat Leg Raises with Arm Circles:** 12 reps each leg.
7. **One-Legged Wall Plank with Leg Lifts:** 12 lifts each leg.
8. **Wall Roll-Downs with Arm Circles:** 10 reps.

Cool Down:

- **Seated Forward Fold:** 1 minute.
- **Shoulder Stretch against Wall:** 30 seconds each arm.

Progressive Wall Pilates Routines

Routine 1: Wall Pilates Foundation

Objective:

Establish basic familiarity with wall-based Pilates movements.

Sequence:

1. **Wall Squats:** 3 sets of 10 reps.
2. **Wall Plank Hold:** 3 sets of 20 seconds.
3. **Wall Angels:** 2 sets of 8 reps.
4. **Wall Push-Ups:** 3 sets of 8 reps.
5. **Wall Roll-Downs:** 2 sets of 6 reps.

Progression:

Increase sets and reps gradually every week for a month. Focus on form and control.

Routine 2: Building Stability

Objective:

Enhance stability and core engagement in wall-based exercises.

Sequence:

1. **Wall Squats with Leg Raises:** 3 sets of 12 reps.
2. **One-Legged Wall Plank Hold:** 3 sets of 15 seconds each leg.
3. **Dynamic Wall Angels:** 2 sets of 10 reps.
4. **Wall Push-Ups with Rotation:** 3 sets of 10 reps.
5. **Wall Roll-Downs with Arm Circles:** 2 sets of 8 reps.

Progression:

Increase hold times for the one-legged wall plank and add small pulses to the dynamic wall angels.

Routine 3: Increasing Endurance

Objective:

Focus on increasing muscular endurance in wall-based exercises.

Sequence:

1. **Wall Squats with Ball Squeeze:** 3 sets of 15 reps.
2. **Wall Plank Leg Lifts:** 3 sets of 12 lifts each leg.
3. **Wall Angels with Resistance Band:** 2 sets of 12 reps.
4. **Decline Wall Push-Ups:** 3 sets of 12 reps.
5. **Wall Roll-Downs with Leg Slide:** 2 sets of 10 reps.

Progression:

Add a hold at the bottom position of wall squats and increase the resistance in wall angels.

Routine 4: Introducing Complexity

Objective:

Incorporate complex movements and variations into the routine.

Sequence:

1. **Wall Squats with Arm Raises and Calf Raises:** 3 sets of 12 reps.
2. **Wall Plank Flow:** 2 continuous flows integrating various variations.
3. **Plyometric Wall Push-Ups:** 3 sets of 10 reps.
4. **Wall Angels with Leg Raises:** 2 sets of 12 reps.
5. **Wall Plank Shoulder Taps with Side Leg Raises:** 3 sets of 10 taps and raises each side.

Progression:

Increase the speed of plyometric wall push-ups and aim for seamless transitions in wall plank flow.

Routine 5: Advanced Strength and Control

Objective:

Develop advanced strength and control in wall-based Pilates exercises.

Sequence:

1. **Wall Squats with Arm Circles and Twist:** 3 sets of 15 reps.
2. **One-Legged Wall Plank with Arm Variations:** 3 sets of 20 seconds each leg.
3. **Wall Angels with Dynamic Pulses:** 2 sets of 15 reps.
4. **Wall Push-Ups with Knee to Elbow:** 3 sets of 12 reps.
5. **Wall Roll-Downs with Side Bends:** 2 sets of 10 reps.

Progression:

Increase the range of motion in wall squats and add a hold at the top of one-legged wall planks.

Routine 6: Progressive Flow and Endurance

Objective:

Focus on a continuous flow of movements while increasing endurance.

Sequence:

1. **Dynamic Wall Squats with Arm Swings:** 3 sets of 15 reps.
2. **Wall Plank Flow with Knee Tucks and Arm Reaches:** 2 rounds.
3. **Plyometric Wall Push-Ups:** 3 sets of 12 reps.
4. **Wall Angels with Resistance Band and Pulses:** 2 sets of 15 reps.
5. **Wall Plank with Shoulder Taps and Leg Lifts:** 3 sets of 10 taps and lifts each side.

Progression:

Strive for fluidity and increase the number of rounds in wall plank flow.

Routine 7: Complex Movements and Balance

Objective:

Integrate complex movements while improving balance.

Sequence:

1. **Wall Squats with Leg Raises and Arm Circles:** 3 sets of 12 reps.
2. **Wall Plank Flow with Twists and Leg Lifts:** 2 rounds.
3. **One-Legged Wall Squats with Arm Reaches:** 3 sets of 10 reps each leg.
4. **Wall Plank with Knee Tucks and Arm Reaches:** 3 sets of 12 reps.
5. **Wall Angels with Dynamic Pulses and Twists:** 2 sets of 15 reps.

Progression:

Increase the range of motion in one-legged wall squats and add twists to wall plank exercises.

Routine 8: Advanced Functional Strength

Objective:

Develop advanced functional strength in wall-based exercises.

Sequence:

1. **Wall Squats with Forward Fold and Toe Touches:** 3 sets of 12 reps.
2. **Wall Plank Flow with Dynamic Knee Tucks and Arm Reaches:** 2 rounds.
3. **Plyometric Wall Push-Ups with Decline:** 3 sets of 12 reps.
4. **Wall Angels with Resistance Band and Leg Raises:** 2 sets of 15 reps.
5. **One-Legged Wall Plank with Dynamic Arm Circles:** 3 sets of 20 seconds each leg.

Progression:

Increase the speed and explosiveness in plyometric wall push-ups and aim for controlled arm movements in one-legged wall planks.

Routine 9: Advanced Flexibility and Stability Fusion

Objective:

Combine advanced flexibility with stability-focused exercises.

Sequence:

1. **Wall Squats with Forward Fold and Leg Swings:** 3 sets of 12 reps.
2. **Wall Plank Flow with Dynamic Leg Lifts and Arm Circles:** 2 rounds.
3. **Dynamic Wall Squats with Arm Swings and Twist:** 3 sets of 15 reps.
4. **Wall Plank with Shoulder Stretches and Rotation:** 3 sets of 10 reps.
5. **One-Legged Wall Plank with Side Stretch and Reach:** 3 sets of 15 seconds each leg.

Progression:

Focus on deeper stretches in wall squats and increase hold times in one-legged wall planks.

Routine 10: Advanced Dynamic Power Circuit

Objective:

Combine dynamic power movements in a circuit.

Circuit (Repeat 3 times):

1. **Plyometric Wall Push-Ups:** 15 reps.
2. **Wall Plank Flow with Knee to Elbow and Leg Lifts:** 12 reps each side.
3. **Wall Squats with Leg Raises and Arm Circles:** 12 reps.
4. **Wall Plank Flow with Arm Reaches and Twists:** 2 rounds.
5. **Wall Squat Leg Raises with Arm Circles:** 12 reps each leg.
6. **One-Legged Wall Plank with Leg Lifts:** 12 lifts each leg.
7. **Wall Roll-Downs with Arm Circles:** 10 reps.

Progression:

Focus on explusiveness and seamless transitions within the circuit.

Addison Mitchell

Chapter 4: Enhancing Your Wall Pilates Practice

Mindfulness and Relaxation

Mindfulness refers to the practice of maintaining a moment-by-moment awareness of thoughts, feelings, bodily sensations, and the surrounding environment, without judgment. It involves being fully present and engaged in the current experience, acknowledging and accepting one's thoughts and feelings without reacting or becoming overwhelmed by them.

In the context of exercise, such as Wall Pilates, mindfulness can be applied by consciously focusing on the movements, the sensations in the body, and the breath. It helps in enhancing the mind-body connection, improving concentration, and fostering a deeper understanding of how different movements affect the body.

Relaxation, on the other hand, refers to the state of being free from tension, stress, or anxiety. It involves consciously releasing physical, mental, and emotional strain. In the context of exercise routines like Wall Pilates, relaxation techniques are integrated into the cooldown phase, aiming to reduce muscle tension, calm the mind, and promote overall well-being.

Combining mindfulness and relaxation techniques in exercise routines like Wall Pilates creates an opportunity to not only strengthen the body but also cultivate mental clarity, reduce stress, and enhance the overall experience of the workout. These techniques encourage practitioners to be fully present in the moment, fostering a sense of calmness and centeredness both during and after the workout session.

Incorporating Mindfulness Techniques

1. **Breath-Centric Awareness:**

   - *Beginning the Practice:* Encourage practitioners to start by focusing on their breath, using it as an anchor throughout the session.
   - *Breath Synchronization:* Guide individuals to sync their breath with movements, emphasizing inhales for expansion and exhales for contraction.

2. **Body Scan and Awareness:**

   - *Starting with Stillness:* Initiate the session by standing against the wall, encouraging practitioners to do a mental check-in from head to toe, noticing areas of tension or relaxation.
   - *Progressive Muscle Engagement:* Encourage gradual muscle engagement, starting from the core and radiating outwards, fostering a heightened sense of body awareness.

3. **Mindful Transitions:**

   - *Focus on Transitions:* Encourage attention during transitions between exercises against the wall, emphasizing smooth and controlled movements.
   - *Intentional Movement:* Urge practitioners to consciously move each body part, maintaining awareness throughout the transition phase.

4. **Mindful Focus during Wall-Based Exercises:**

   - *Engaging Concentration:* Encourage a laser-like focus on the muscles being targeted during each wall-based movement.

- *Quality over Quantity:* Emphasize the importance of precision and form, valuing controlled movements over speed.

5. Integrating Breath with Movement:

- *Flowing with Breath:* Encourage individuals to let the breath guide their movements, creating a harmonious connection between breath and motion.

- *Mindful Expansion and Contraction:* Highlight the sensation of muscles expanding during inhalation and contracting during exhalation while performing wall Pilates exercises.

6. Mindful Cooldown and Relaxation:

- *Transition to Calm:* Initiate the cooldown phase by guiding practitioners through slow movements against the wall, emphasizing relaxation and release of tension.

- *Deep Breathing Techniques:* Incorporate deep breathing exercises against the wall, focusing on elongated exhalations to promote relaxation.

7. Mindful Visualization and Meditation:

- *Visual Imagery:* Offer visual cues to enhance mind-body connection, encouraging individuals to visualize muscles engaging and releasing with each movement against the wall.

- *Guided Meditation:* Conclude the routine with a brief guided meditation, focusing on gratitude and a sense of accomplishment from the practice.

8. Mindfulness beyond the Wall:

- *Daily Application:* Encourage practitioners to carry mindfulness beyond the wall, applying techniques like conscious breathing and body awareness in their daily routines.

- *Mindful Living:* Emphasize the incorporation of mindfulness principles into everyday activities, fostering a sense of mindfulness in all aspects of life.

Cooling Down with Wall Pilates

1. **Transitioning from Intensity:**
   - *Gradual Decrease in Intensity:* After completing the main wall-based exercises, gradually reduce the intensity of movements.
   - *Slower Pace:* Shift from dynamic movements against the wall to slower, controlled motions.

2. **Focus on Breathing and Relaxation:**
   - *Breath Awareness:* Emphasize deep, intentional breathing, guiding practitioners to inhale deeply and exhale fully.
   - *Mindful Relaxation:* Encourage a mindful approach, inviting individuals to relax the muscles engaged during the workout against the wall.

3. **Static Stretches against the Wall:**
   - *Targeted Stretches:* Perform static stretches against the wall, focusing on major muscle groups engaged during the workout.
   - *Hold and Release:* Hold each stretch for around 15-30 seconds, allowing the muscles to lengthen, then release gradually.

4. **Emphasizing Flexibility:**
   - *Increasing Range of Motion:* Use the wall to aid in deepening stretches, enhancing flexibility.
   - *Full-Body Stretching:* Include stretches targeting the upper body, lower body, back, and shoulders against the wall.

Addison Mitchell

5. Mindful Mind-Body Connection:

- *Attention to Sensations:* Encourage practitioners to pay attention to the sensations in the body during stretches, fostering a deeper mind-body connection.

- *Relaxing Tight Muscles:* Emphasize breathing into tight areas to promote relaxation and release tension.

6. Promoting Recovery:

- *Facilitating Recovery:* Cooling down with Wall Pilates helps reduce muscle soreness and stiffness post-workout.

- *Enhancing Circulation:* Encourage gentle movements to aid in the distribution of blood flow and nutrients to tired muscles.

7. Mindful Closure of the Session:

- *Reflective Closure:* Conclude the cooling down phase with a moment of reflection, acknowledging the effort put into the workout.

- *Expressing Gratitude:* Invite individuals to express gratitude for the practice and their bodies.

8. Transition to Post-Workout Relaxation:

- *Seamless Transition:* Use the cooling down phase as a bridge to post-workout relaxation techniques, such as deep breathing or guided meditation.

- *Preparation for Recovery:* Set the stage for the body to enter a state of rest and recovery after the Wall Pilates session.

Optimizing Your Wall Pilates Journey

1. **Setting Realistic Goals:**

   - *Goal Identification:* Encourage practitioners to define specific, achievable goals aligned with their fitness aspirations.
   - *Long-term Vision*

2. **Consistency and Commitment:**

   - *Regular Practice:* Emphasize the significance of consistent practice in reaping the benefits of Wall Pilates.
   - *Establishing Routine*

3. **Mindful Progress Tracking:**

   - *Journaling Progress:* Encourage keeping a workout journal to track improvements in strength, flexibility, and overall performance in Wall Pilates exercises.
   - *Revisiting Goals:* Periodically review and adjust goals based on progress made in the Wall Pilates journey.

4. **Proper Technique Emphasis:**

   - *Focus on Form.*
   - *Seeking Guidance:* Encourage seeking guidance from certified instructors to ensure correct posture and execution.

5. Progressive Challenge and Variation:

- *Gradual Intensity Increase*
- *Variety in Practice:* Encourage the inclusion of diverse exercises and sequences against the wall to target different muscle groups and avoid plateauing.

6. Rest and Recovery:

- *Understanding Recovery:* Stress the importance of adequate rest and recovery periods between Wall Pilates sessions for muscle repair and growth.
- *Balancing Intensity.*

7. Nutrition and Hydration:

- *Fueling the Body*
- *Hydration Importance:* Emphasize staying hydrated to optimize performance and aid in muscle recovery.

8. Mind-Body Connection:

- *Breath Awareness:* Encourage practitioners to focus on synchronized breathing with movements against the wall, enhancing the mind-body connection.
- *Mental Focus*

9. Adaptability and Patience:

- *Embracing Adaptation*
- *Patience in Progress:* Encourage patience and persistence, acknowledging that progress in Wall Pilates is gradual and varies for each individual.

10. **Celebrating Milestones:**

- *Acknowledging Achievements:* Encourage celebrating milestones and successes reached in the Wall Pilates journey, fostering motivation and a sense of accomplishment.

- *Encouraging Community:* Suggest joining communities or classes to share experiences and celebrate collective achievements.

Tips for Long-Term Commitment

1. Establish Clear Goals:

- **Specific Objectives:** Define precise and achievable goals within Wall Pilates, whether it's improving flexibility, building core strength, or enhancing overall fitness.

- **Long-Term Vision:** Create a vision of where you want to be in your Wall Pilates practice, ensuring your goals align with this overarching vision.

2. Cultivate Consistent Practice:

- **Routine Integration:** Make Wall Pilates a regular part of your schedule, allocating fixed days or times for practice.

- **Start Slow, Build Up:** Begin with manageable sessions and gradually increase the frequency and duration as your comfort and proficiency grow.

3. Monitor Progress:

- **Tracking Tools:** Maintain a workout journal or use apps to record progress, note improvements, and track achievements during your Wall Pilates journey.

- **Regular Assessment:** Periodically review your progress against set goals, allowing adjustments and celebrating milestones.

4. Emphasize Technique and Form:

- **Quality Over Quantity:** Focus on proper form and technique in each Wall Pilates exercise, ensuring correct posture and alignment to maximize effectiveness.
- **Seek Guidance:** Consider consulting certified instructors or trainers for guidance on form correction and exercise variations.

5. Gradual Challenge and Variety:

- **Progressive Intensity:** Gradually increase the difficulty or intensity of your Wall Pilates exercises to avoid plateaus and sustain continuous improvement.
- **Mix It Up:** Incorporate diverse exercises, sequences, or variations to engage different muscle groups and keep your practice fresh and interesting.

6. Prioritize Recovery:

- **Rest Periods:** Allow sufficient time for rest and recovery between Wall Pilates sessions to prevent fatigue and promote muscle repair.
- **Restorative Practices:** Integrate stretching, relaxation, and activities that aid in muscle recovery to balance out intense workouts.

7. Balanced Lifestyle:

- **Nutrition:** Maintain a balanced diet that supports your energy needs for Wall Pilates workouts and aids in recovery.
- **Hydration:** Ensure adequate hydration to optimize performance, aid recovery, and sustain overall well-being.

8. Nurture Mind-Body Connection:

- **Breath Awareness:** Practice synchronized breathing with movements against the wall, enhancing coordination and mindfulness during exercises.

- **Mental Focus:** Engage your mind in the practice, concentrating on muscle engagement and movement precision.

9. Adaptability and Persistence:

- **Flexibility in Approach:** Adapt Wall Pilates exercises to your fitness level and listen to your body, allowing modifications when necessary.
- **Patience and Persistence:** Understand that progress takes time; stay patient and committed to your practice, acknowledging small victories along the way.

10. Community and Support:

- **Join Communities:** Engage with fellow practitioners or classes to share experiences, seek advice, and draw inspiration from a supportive community.
- **Accountability Partner:** Consider partnering with someone to keep each other motivated and accountable in your Wall Pilates journey.

By incorporating these strategies into your Wall Pilates routine, you can cultivate a sustainable and fulfilling long-term commitment, ensuring consistent progress and overall well-being.

BONUS: 28 DAY CHALLENGE

This 28-day challenge offers a structured progression through fundamental exercises, gradually escalating to more advanced routines, encouraging consistency, technique refinement, and skill development in Wall Pilates workouts. Adjust repetitions, sets, and exercises as needed to suit individual fitness levels and goals.

Week 1: Foundation Building

Days 1-7: Focus on Fundamentals

- **Day 1:** Begin with Wall Squats and Wall Push-Ups - 3 sets of 10 reps each.
- **Day 3:** Introduce Wall Roll-Downs and Wall Angels - 2 sets of 8 reps each.
- **Day 5:** Practice Wall Planks and Wall Pilates Routines 1 & 2.
- **Day 7:** Review exercises from the week; aim for 20 minutes of continuous Wall Pilates flow.

Week 2: Increasing Intensity

Days 8-14: Progressive Workouts

- **Day 8-10:** Increase sets to 4 and reps to 12 for Wall Squats and Push-Ups.
- **Day 12-14:** Perform 3 sets of 10 reps for Wall Roll-Down Variations and Wall Angels.
- **Day 14:** Engage in Wall Pilates Routines 3 & 4, incorporating a 25-minute continuous flow.

Week 3: Diversification and Challenge

Days 15-21: Varied Exercises and Sequences

- **Day 15-17:** Try Challenging Wall Pilates Sequences 1 & 2 - 2 sets of 8 reps each.
- **Day 19-21:** Experiment with 3 sets of 10 reps for Wall Plank Variations and Wall Pilates Routines 5 & 6.
- **Day 21:** Create a personalized sequence using any Wall Pilates exercises; aim for a 30-minute uninterrupted session.

Week 4: Mastery and Finale

Days 22-28: Advanced and Mastery

- **Day 22-24:** Advance to Advanced Wall Pilates Workouts 1 & 2 - 3 sets of 10 reps.
- **Day 26-28:** Perform 2 sets of 12 reps for Wall Pilates Routines 7 & 8, focusing on smooth transitions and fluidity.
- **Day 28:** Challenge yourself with Wall Pilates Routines 9 & 10, aiming for a 40-minute session showcasing your acquired mastery.

Meet the Author: Addison Mitchell

Exploring the Author's Insights:

Discover more about Addison Mitchell's background, insights, and journey in health and culinary wellness through her Amazon Author Central page. Click the link or scan the QR code below to dive deeper into the author's profile, exploring an array of informative articles, author updates, and additional resources related to fitness, health, wellness, and culinary solutions.

Explore these captivating works by Addison Mitchell, each offering unique perspectives on fitness, wall Pilates, yoga, health, wellness, and many more for seniors, beginners, women, men, women over 50 and lots of category. Visit the Amazon Author Central page to access more captivating reads and engage with the author's enriching content.

YOU CAN FOLLOW ACCOUNT SO YOU GET NOTIFIED WHEN WE DROP UPDATED AND NEW WORKOUTS BOOK ON GOOD HEALTH.

CLICK LINK BELOW

amazon.com/author/addisonmitchell

OR

SCAN QR CODE TO VIEW

Other works by Addison Mitchell

Explore beyond "Quick and simple wall Pilates workouts" and delve into Addison Mitchell's diverse collection of wall Pilates, encompassing a range of fitness-centric topics and good body adventures. Here is one captivating book authored by Addison Mitchell

1. **WALL PILATES WORKOUTS for seniors over 60**: Illustrated Step-by-Step Workouts Bible for Women, men and beginners Over 60 with Low-Impact Wall Pilates, and Strength Training to lose weight

   ☆☆ ARE YOU A BUSY LADY, OVERWEIGHT PERSON, OR JUST AN OLDER PERSON WHO WISHES TO CONTINUE LIVING AN ACTIVE LIFE? OR ARE YOU GOING THROUGH MENOPAUSE AND ABOVE 50? YOU'RE AT THE CORRECT SPOT, HOWEVER! ☆☆

Unlock the transformative power of fitness with our comprehensive guide, tailor-made for women, men, and beginners over 60 seeking to rejuvenate their health and vitality. In "Illustrated Step-by-Step Workouts Bible for Women, Men, and Beginners Over 60," discover the holistic approach to fitness through Low-Impact Wall Pilates, Chair Yoga, and Strength Training.

CLICK ON THE LINK BELOW TO VIEW

https://www.amazon.com/dp/B0CRJ312NJ

OR

SCAN THE QR CODE TO VIEW

Conclusion

Embarking on the Quick and Simple Wall Pilates Workouts journey unveils a holistic approach to fitness, combining mindful movement, focused breathing, and a dedication to self-improvement. This comprehensive guide is designed to empower individuals seeking to enhance their physical well-being through Wall Pilates exercises. By delving into the depths of this practice, you've ventured into a realm where strength, flexibility, and mindfulness converge to redefine your fitness journey.

Throughout this guide, we've explored various facets critical to mastering Wall Pilates, from the foundational principles to the intricacies of technique, from optimizing progress to nurturing a long-term commitment. Let's recap the pivotal elements uncovered:

Foundational Insights:

- **Table of Contents:** An organized roadmap guiding you through a structured approach to Wall Pilates workouts.
- **Wall Pilates Fundamentals:** Aligning posture, engaging the core, and utilizing the wall for support form the bedrock of these exercises.

Essential Knowledge:

- **Breathing Techniques:** Synchronized breathwork enhancing the mind-body connection during Wall Pilates.
- **Mindfulness and Relaxation:** Elevating workouts by integrating mindful practices and relaxation techniques.
- **Safety Measures:** Prioritizing safety and precautionary measures throughout your Wall Pilates journey.

Comprehensive Practices:

- **Variations and Sequences:** Over 30 varied Wall Pilates exercises and sequences to challenge and diversify your practice.
- **Progressive Routines:** Ten meticulously crafted progressive routines, tailored to advance your skills methodically.

Optimizing Your Journey:

- **Long-Term Commitment:** Tips and strategies encouraging consistency, technique refinement, and adaptation for sustained progress.
- **Mind-Body Connection:** Nurturing the synchronization between breath, movement, and mental focus.
- **Community and Support:** Embracing a sense of community, accountability, and celebration in your journey.

The beauty of Wall Pilates lies not only in the physical transformation it offers but also in the mental fortitude it cultivates. By committing to these quick and simple workouts, you've embarked on a path toward a healthier, stronger, and more centered self. Your journey is unique, and each step, each wall-based movement, contributes to your growth and well-being.

Embrace the challenges, celebrate your achievements, and stay committed to the transformative power of Wall Pilates. May this guide serve as your constant companion, inspiring you to push boundaries, find balance, and evolve on your Wall Pilates journey. As you continue, remember, it's not just about the workout; it's about nurturing a lifestyle of holistic well-being.

With each session against the wall, you embrace the opportunity to redefine your strength, connect with your body, and unfold the potential within. Welcome to a journey of discovery, empowerment, and lasting vitality through Quick and Simple Wall Pilates Workouts.

Thanking Readers and Contributors

To our Valued Readers,

As we bring this comprehensive guide on Quick and Simple Wall Pilates Workouts to a close, our hearts overflow with gratitude for your unwavering dedication and enthusiasm in exploring the transformative world of Wall Pilates. Your commitment to self-improvement and holistic well-being inspires us and fuels the essence of this guide.

We extend our deepest gratitude to each reader who has embarked on this journey, embracing the principles, techniques, and exercises detailed within these pages. Your eagerness to learn, grow, and evolve in your fitness pursuits is truly commendable.

We also wish to express our heartfelt appreciation to the contributors, mentors, and experts whose wisdom, insights, and expertise have enriched this guide. Your dedication to sharing knowledge and enhancing the Wall Pilates experience has been invaluable in shaping this comprehensive resource.

To the vibrant community surrounding Wall Pilates, your support, engagement, and shared experiences have contributed immensely to the nurturing environment of learning and growth.

Remember, your commitment to wellness is a profound testament to your strength and determination. Whether you're starting this journey, have been practicing Wall Pilates for a while, or are an expert in the field, your presence and dedication have played an integral role in making this guide a cornerstone for fitness enthusiasts.

Addison Mitchell

As you continue on your Wall Pilates journey, may the guidance and insights from this resource empower you, the camaraderie of fellow practitioners uplift you, and the transformative power of these workouts invigorate your body, mind, and spirit.

Thank you for being an integral part of this incredible community dedicated to health, vitality, and self-discovery through Wall Pilates.

With deepest gratitude and warmest regards,

[Addison Mitchell]

Printed in the USA
CPSIA information can be obtained
at www.ICGtesting.com
LVHW082157050324
773680LV00040B/1412